FAST FEAST

PROTOCOL RECIPES

28-Day Meal Plans for Building Immune System and Weight Loss Nutrition for Beginners.

Kelvin Himman

Copyright © 2024 by Kelvin Himman

TABLE OF CONTENT

INTRODUCTION

Welcome to "Fast Feast Protocol Recipes: 28-Day Meal Plans for Effortless Immune Support and Weight Loss Nutrition for Beginners." In today's fast-paced world, achieving optimal health and maintaining a healthy weight can feel like an elusive goal.

With countless diet trends and conflicting nutrition advice, it's easy to feel overwhelmed and unsure of where to start.

But what if there was a simple, science-backed approach to nutrition that not only supported your immune system but also helped you shed those stubborn pounds effortlessly? That's where the Fast Feast Protocol comes in.

This revolutionary approach to eating combines the power of intermittent fasting with delicious, nutrient-rich recipes to help you achieve your health and weight loss goals without deprivation or restriction.

In this book, we'll guide you through the principles of the Fast Feast Protocol and provide you with everything you need to embark on a transformative 28-day journey to better health and vitality.

From expert guidance and meticulously crafted meal plans to mouthwatering recipes and practical tips, you'll have all the tools and resources you need to succeed.

Whether you're new to intermittent fasting or looking to take your health and wellness journey to the next level, "Fast Feast Protocol Recipes" is your ultimate companion on the path to a healthier, happier you.

Get ready to experience increased energy, improved digestion, enhanced mental clarity, and a leaner, stronger body—all while enjoying delicious, nourishing meals every step of the way.

Are you ready to unlock the secret to effortless immune support and weight loss? Let's dive in and discover the transformative power of the Fast Feast Protocol together!

Coconut Curry Chicken

Ingredients:

- 1 lb (450g) chicken breast, cut into bite-sized pieces

- 1 tablespoon coconut oil

- 1 onion, diced

- 3 cloves garlic, minced

- 2 tablespoons curry powder

- 1 can (14 oz/400ml) coconut milk

- 1 can (14 oz/400g) diced tomatoes

- 2 cups (120g) fresh spinach leaves

- Salt and pepper to taste

- Cooked cauliflower rice or regular rice, for serving

- Fresh cilantro, chopped (optional, for garnish)

Preparation:

1. **Sauté Chicken:** In a large skillet, heat coconut oil over medium heat. Add diced chicken pieces and cook until they're browned on all sides, about 5-7 minutes.

Remove the chicken from the skillet and set aside.

2. **Sauté Aromatics:** In the same skillet, add diced onion and minced garlic. Sauté until onions are translucent and garlic is fragrant, about 2-3 minutes.

3. **Add Curry Powder:** Sprinkle curry powder over the onion and garlic mixture. Stir well to coat the aromatics with the curry powder.

4. **Simmer with Coconut Milk:** Pour in the coconut milk and diced tomatoes. Stir to combine everything. Bring the mixture to a simmer.

5. **Return Chicken:** Return the cooked chicken to the skillet. Stir to combine with the coconut curry sauce. Let it simmer for another 10-15 minutes until the chicken is cooked through and the sauce has thickened slightly.

6. **Add Spinach:** Once the chicken is cooked, add fresh spinach leaves to the skillet. Stir until the spinach wilts and incorporates into the curry sauce.

7. **Season and Serve:** Taste the curry and season with salt and pepper according to

your preference. Serve the coconut curry chicken over cooked cauliflower rice or regular rice. Garnish with chopped cilantro if desired.

Benefits:

- **Protein Source:** Chicken breast provides a lean source of protein, essential for muscle repair and growth.

- **Healthy Fats:** Coconut milk offers healthy fats, particularly medium-chain triglycerides (MCTs), which can provide a quick source of energy and may aid in weight loss.

- **Immune Support:** Garlic and onion contain compounds that can support immune function and overall health.

- **Antioxidants:** Spinach is rich in antioxidants like vitamin C and beta-carotene, which help protect cells from damage caused by free radicals.

- **Anti-inflammatory:** Turmeric, often found in curry powder, contains curcumin, known for its anti-inflammatory properties.

- **Vitamins and Minerals:** This dish provides essential vitamins and minerals from various ingredients, contributing to overall health and well-being.

Tofu Veggie Stir-Fry

Ingredients:

- 14 oz (400g) firm tofu, pressed and cubed
- 2 tablespoons soy sauce
- 1 tablespoon sesame oil
- 1 tablespoon cornstarch
- 2 tablespoons vegetable oil
- 2 cloves garlic, minced
- 1 teaspoon grated ginger
- 1 bell pepper, sliced
- 1 cup (150g) snap peas, trimmed
- 1 carrot, julienned
- 1 cup (120g) broccoli florets
- 2 green onions, sliced
- Cooked brown rice or quinoa, for serving
- Sesame seeds (optional, for garnish)

Preparation:

1. **Prepare Tofu:** In a bowl, combine cubed tofu with soy sauce, sesame oil, and

cornstarch. Toss gently to coat the tofu evenly.

2. **Sauté Tofu:** Heat vegetable oil in a large skillet or wok over medium-high heat. Add the marinated tofu cubes and cook until golden brown on all sides, about 5-7 minutes. Remove tofu from the skillet and set aside.

3. **Sauté Aromatics:** In the same skillet, add minced garlic and grated ginger. Sauté for about 1 minute until fragrant.

4. **Add Vegetables:** Add sliced bell pepper, snap peas, julienned carrot, and broccoli florets to the skillet. Stir-fry for 3-4 minutes until the vegetables are tender-crisp.

5. **Combine Tofu:** Return the cooked tofu to the skillet with the vegetables. Toss everything together until heated through.

6. **Finish and Serve:** Sprinkle sliced green onions over the stir-fry. Serve the tofu and veggie stir-fry hot over cooked brown rice or quinoa. Garnish with sesame seeds if desired.

Benefits:

- **Protein Source:** Tofu provides a plant-based source of protein, making this dish suitable for vegetarians and vegans.

- **Healthy Fats:** Sesame oil offers healthy fats and adds a nutty flavor to the stir-fry.

- **Fiber and Nutrients:** The variety of vegetables in this stir-fry, including bell pepper, snap peas, carrot, and broccoli, provide fiber, vitamins, and minerals essential for overall health.

- **Low in Calories:** This dish is low in calories but high in nutrient density, making it suitable for weight management and promoting satiety.

- **Quick and Easy:** Stir-fries are quick to prepare and cook, making them perfect for busy weeknights when you want a healthy meal on the table fast.

- **Customizable:** You can easily customize this stir-fry by adding your favorite vegetables or adjusting the seasonings to suit your taste preferences.

Vegetable Egg Muffins

Ingredients:

- 6 large eggs

- 1/4 cup milk (dairy or non-dairy)

- 1 cup mixed vegetables (such as spinach, bell peppers, onions, tomatoes, mushrooms), chopped

- 1/2 cup shredded cheese (cheddar, mozzarella, or your favorite cheese)

- Salt and pepper, to taste

- Cooking spray or olive oil, for greasing muffin tin

Preparation:

1. **Preheat Oven:** Preheat your oven to 350°F (175°C). Grease a 6-cup muffin tin with cooking spray or olive oil.

2. **Prepare Eggs:** In a large mixing bowl, crack the eggs and whisk them together with the milk until well combined. Season with salt and pepper to taste.

3. **Add Vegetables:** Stir in the chopped mixed vegetables of your choice into the

egg mixture. Make sure the vegetables are evenly distributed.

4. **Fill Muffin Tin:** Pour the egg and vegetable mixture evenly into the greased muffin tin, filling each cup about 3/4 full.

5. **Add Cheese:** Sprinkle shredded cheese over the top of each egg muffin cup, distributing it evenly.

6. **Bake:** Place the muffin tin in the preheated oven and bake for 20-25 minutes, or until the egg muffins are set and the tops are golden brown.

7. **Cool and Serve:** Remove the egg muffins from the oven and let them cool in the muffin tin for a few minutes. Use a knife to loosen the edges, then carefully remove the egg muffins from the tin. Serve warm or at room temperature.

Benefits:

- **High in Protein:** Eggs are a rich source of high-quality protein, essential for muscle repair and growth.

- **Vegetable-Rich:** These egg muffins are packed with a variety of vegetables, providing essential vitamins, minerals, and dietary fiber.

- **Customizable:** You can easily customize these egg muffins by using your favorite vegetables or adding cooked meats like bacon or sausage.

- **Portable and Convenient:** Vegetable egg muffins are perfect for meal prep and on-the-go breakfasts or snacks. They can be stored in the refrigerator and reheated quickly in the microwave.

- **Low in Carbs:** These egg muffins are naturally low in carbohydrates, making them suitable for low-carb or ketogenic diets.

- **Versatile:** You can enjoy these vegetable egg muffins as they are or serve them with a side of whole-grain toast, fresh fruit, or a salad for a complete meal. They're also great for adding protein and veggies to lunch or dinner.

Lemon Garlic Shrimp Skewers

Ingredients:

- 1 lb (450g) large shrimp, peeled and deveined

- 3 cloves garlic, minced

- Zest and juice of 1 lemon

- 2 tablespoons olive oil

- 1 tablespoon chopped fresh parsley

- Salt and pepper, to taste

- Wooden or metal skewers

Preparation:

1. **Marinate Shrimp:** In a bowl, combine minced garlic, lemon zest, lemon juice, olive oil, chopped parsley, salt, and pepper. Add the peeled and deveined shrimp to the bowl and toss to coat evenly. Let the shrimp marinate for at least 15-30 minutes in the refrigerator.

2. **Preheat Grill:** If using wooden skewers, soak them in water for about 30 minutes to prevent burning. Preheat your grill to medium-high heat.

3. **Skewer Shrimp:** Thread the marinated shrimp onto skewers, dividing them evenly.

4. **Grill Shrimp:** Place the shrimp skewers on the preheated grill. Cook for 2-3 minutes on each side, or until the shrimp are pink and opaque.

5. **Serve:** Once the shrimp are cooked through, remove them from the grill and transfer to a serving platter. Garnish with additional chopped parsley and lemon wedges if desired. Serve hot.

Benefits:

- **High Protein:** Shrimp is a lean source of protein, providing essential amino acids necessary for muscle repair and growth.

- **Healthy Fats:** Olive oil used in the marinade adds healthy monounsaturated fats, which are beneficial for heart health.

- **Vitamin C:** Lemon juice not only adds flavor but also provides a boost of vitamin C, an antioxidant that supports immune function and skin health.

- **Low in Calories:** Shrimp is relatively low in calories and fat, making it a suitable option for those watching their calorie intake.

- **Quick and Easy:** This recipe comes together quickly and is perfect for busy weeknights or outdoor grilling sessions.

- **Versatile:** Lemon garlic shrimp skewers can be served as an appetizer, main dish, or added to salads, pasta, or rice dishes for extra protein and flavor.

- **Delicious and Flavorful:** The combination of garlic, lemon, and fresh herbs infuses the shrimp with bright, zesty flavors that are sure to please your taste buds.

Broccoli and Chicken Stir-Fry

Ingredients:

- 1 lb (450g) boneless, skinless chicken breasts, thinly sliced

- 2 cups (200g) broccoli florets

- 1 red bell pepper, thinly sliced

- 1 yellow bell pepper, thinly sliced

- 1 carrot, julienned

- 3 cloves garlic, minced

- 1 tablespoon fresh ginger, grated

- 2 tablespoons soy sauce

- 1 tablespoon oyster sauce

- 1 tablespoon cornstarch

- 2 tablespoons vegetable oil

- Cooked rice or noodles, for serving

- Sesame seeds and sliced green onions, for garnish (optional)

Preparation:

1. **Marinate Chicken:** In a bowl, combine thinly sliced chicken breast with minced garlic, grated ginger, soy sauce, oyster

sauce, and cornstarch. Stir well to coat the chicken evenly. Let it marinate for at least 15-30 minutes.

2. **Blanch Broccoli:** Bring a pot of water to a boil. Add broccoli florets and blanch for 1-2 minutes, then immediately transfer them to a bowl of ice water to stop the cooking process. Drain and set aside.

3. **Stir-Fry Chicken:** Heat vegetable oil in a large skillet or wok over medium-high heat. Add the marinated chicken and stir-fry for 4-5 minutes until cooked through and no longer pink. Remove the chicken from the skillet and set aside.

4. **Cook Vegetables:** In the same skillet, add sliced bell peppers and julienned carrot. Stir-fry for 2-3 minutes until they start to soften.

5. **Combine Ingredients:** Return the cooked chicken to the skillet with the vegetables. Add blanched broccoli florets. Stir everything together and cook for an additional 2-3 minutes until heated through.

6. **Serve:** Serve the broccoli and chicken stir-fry hot over cooked rice or noodles.

Garnish with sesame seeds and sliced green onions if desired.

Benefits:

- **Lean Protein:** Chicken breast is a lean source of protein, essential for muscle repair and growth.

- **Fiber and Nutrients:** Broccoli, bell peppers, and carrots are rich in fiber, vitamins, and minerals, contributing to overall health and well-being.

- **Low in Calories:** This stir-fry is low in calories but high in nutrient density, making it suitable for weight management and promoting satiety.

- **Quick and Easy:** Stir-fries come together quickly and are perfect for busy weeknights when you want a healthy meal on the table fast.

- **Customizable:** You can easily customize this stir-fry by adding your favorite vegetables or adjusting the seasonings to suit your taste preferences.

- **Versatile:** Serve this broccoli and chicken stir-fry over rice, noodles, or quinoa for a complete meal. Leftovers can be enjoyed for lunch the next day or repurposed into wraps, salads, or grain bowls.

Caprese Quinoa Salad

Ingredients:

- 1 cup quinoa
- 2 cups water or vegetable broth
- 1 pint cherry tomatoes, halved
- 1 ball fresh mozzarella cheese, diced
- 1/4 cup fresh basil leaves, thinly sliced
- 2 tablespoons extra virgin olive oil
- 1 tablespoon balsamic glaze or balsamic vinegar
- Salt and pepper, to taste

Preparation:

1. **Rinse Quinoa:** Rinse the quinoa under cold water in a fine-mesh strainer to remove any bitterness.

2. **Cook Quinoa:** In a saucepan, combine the rinsed quinoa and water or vegetable broth. Bring to a boil, then reduce heat to low, cover, and simmer for 15-20 minutes, or until the quinoa is cooked and the liquid is absorbed. Remove from heat and let it sit covered for 5 minutes. Fluff with a fork and let it cool.

3. **Assemble Salad:** In a large mixing bowl, combine the cooked quinoa, halved cherry tomatoes, diced fresh mozzarella, and thinly sliced basil leaves.

4. **Dress Salad:** Drizzle extra virgin olive oil and balsamic glaze (or balsamic vinegar) over the salad ingredients. Season with salt and pepper to taste.

5. **Toss and Serve:** Gently toss all the ingredients together until well combined. Taste and adjust seasoning if necessary.

6. **Chill and Serve:** Refrigerate the Caprese quinoa salad for at least 30 minutes to allow the flavors to meld together. Serve chilled or at room temperature.

Benefits:

- **Complete Protein:** Quinoa is a complete protein, containing all nine essential amino acids, making this salad a nutritious option for vegetarians and vegans.

- **Antioxidants:** Cherry tomatoes and basil are rich in antioxidants, which help protect cells from damage caused by free radicals and contribute to overall health.

- **Calcium and Protein:** Fresh mozzarella cheese provides calcium and additional protein, important for bone health and muscle repair.

- **Heart-Healthy Fats:** Extra virgin olive oil offers heart-healthy monounsaturated fats, which can help lower cholesterol levels and reduce the risk of heart disease.

- **Fiber and Nutrients:** This salad is packed with fiber, vitamins, and minerals from the quinoa, tomatoes, and basil, supporting digestive health and overall well-being.

- **Low in Calories:** Caprese quinoa salad is low in calories but high in nutrient density, making it suitable for weight management and promoting satiety.

- **Versatile:** You can customize this salad by adding additional ingredients such as avocado, arugula, or pine nuts for extra flavor and texture. It can also be served as a side dish or a light main course.

Cabbage and Turkey Sauté

Ingredients:

- 1 lb (450g) ground turkey
- 1 small head cabbage, thinly sliced
- 1 onion, thinly sliced
- 2 cloves garlic, minced
- 1 tablespoon olive oil
- 1 tablespoon soy sauce (or tamari for gluten-free option)
- 1 teaspoon ground ginger
- Salt and pepper, to taste
- Sesame seeds and chopped green onions, for garnish (optional)

Preparation:

1. **Cook Turkey:** Heat olive oil in a large skillet or wok over medium-high heat. Add ground turkey to the skillet and cook, breaking it apart with a spatula, until it is browned and cooked through, about 5-7 minutes. Remove the cooked turkey from the skillet and set aside.

2. **Sauté Vegetables:** In the same skillet, add sliced onion and minced garlic. Sauté for 2-3 minutes until the onion is softened and translucent.

3. **Add Cabbage:** Add thinly sliced cabbage to the skillet with the onion and garlic. Stir well to combine.

4. **Season and Cook:** Sprinkle ground ginger over the cabbage mixture. Drizzle soy sauce (or tamari) over the cabbage. Season with salt and pepper to taste. Stir everything together and cook for 5-7 minutes, or until the cabbage is tender but still slightly crisp.

5. **Combine with Turkey:** Return the cooked turkey to the skillet with the cabbage mixture. Stir well to combine and heat through for another 2-3 minutes.

6. **Serve:** Transfer the cabbage and turkey sauté to a serving dish. Garnish with sesame seeds and chopped green onions if desired.

Benefits:

- **Lean Protein:** Ground turkey provides a lean source of protein, essential for muscle repair and growth.

- **Fiber and Nutrients:** Cabbage is rich in fiber, vitamins (especially vitamin C), and minerals, supporting digestive health, immune function, and overall well-being.

- **Low in Calories:** Cabbage and turkey sauté is low in calories but high in nutrient density, making it suitable for weight management and promoting satiety.

- **Heart-Healthy Fats:** Olive oil used for sautéing adds heart-healthy monounsaturated fats, which can help lower cholesterol levels and reduce the risk of heart disease.

- **Quick and Easy:** This recipe comes together quickly and is perfect for busy weeknights when you want a healthy meal on the table fast.

- **Versatile:** You can customize this sauté by adding additional vegetables such as bell peppers, carrots, or mushrooms for extra flavor and nutrition. It can also be served over brown rice, quinoa, or cauliflower rice for a complete meal.

Tuna Salad Lettuce Wraps

Ingredients:

- 2 cans (5 oz each) of tuna in water, drained
- 1/4 cup Greek yogurt
- 1/4 cup diced celery
- 2 tablespoons diced red onion
- 1 tablespoon lemon juice
- 1 tablespoon Dijon mustard
- Salt and pepper, to taste
- Lettuce leaves (such as romaine or butter lettuce) for wrapping
- Sliced cucumber and tomato for garnish (optional)

Preparation:

1. **Prepare Tuna Salad:** In a mixing bowl, combine drained tuna, Greek yogurt, diced celery, diced red onion, lemon juice, and Dijon mustard. Mix well until all ingredients are evenly combined.

2. **Season:** Season the tuna salad with salt and pepper to taste. Adjust the amount of seasoning according to your preference.

3. **Assemble Lettuce Wraps:** Lay out lettuce leaves on a clean surface. Spoon a portion of the tuna salad mixture onto each lettuce leaf.

4. **Garnish:** Optionally, garnish each lettuce wrap with sliced cucumber and tomato for added freshness and crunch.

5. **Wrap and Serve:** Roll up the lettuce leaves around the tuna salad filling, creating wraps. Secure with toothpicks if necessary.

6. **Serve:** Arrange the tuna salad lettuce wraps on a serving platter and serve immediately.

Benefits:

- **High in Protein:** Tuna is a rich source of protein, which is essential for muscle repair and growth.

- **Low in Calories:** This recipe is low in calories, making it suitable for those watching their calorie intake or trying to lose weight.

- **Healthy Fats:** Tuna contains omega-3 fatty acids, which are beneficial for heart health and brain function.

- **Rich in Vitamins and Minerals:** Tuna is a good source of various vitamins and minerals, including vitamin D, vitamin B12, selenium, and iodine.

- **Low Carb Option:** Lettuce wraps are a low-carb alternative to traditional wraps or sandwiches, making them suitable for low-carb or ketogenic diets.

- **Quick and Easy:** This recipe is quick and easy to prepare, making it perfect for busy weeknights or as a quick lunch option.

- **Customizable:** You can customize the tuna salad mixture by adding additional ingredients such as chopped pickles, avocado, or herbs according to your taste preferences.

- **Portable:** Tuna salad lettuce wraps are portable and can be packed for lunch or enjoyed as a snack on the go. They are also a great option for picnics or outdoor gatherings.

Black Bean and Sweet Potato Tacos

Ingredients:

- 2 medium sweet potatoes, peeled and diced
- 1 can (15 oz) black beans, drained and rinsed
- 1 tablespoon olive oil
- 1 teaspoon ground cumin
- 1 teaspoon chili powder
- 1/2 teaspoon paprika
- Salt and pepper, to taste
- 8 small corn or flour tortillas
- Toppings: diced avocado, salsa, shredded lettuce, chopped cilantro, lime wedges

Preparation:

1. **Roast Sweet Potatoes:** Preheat your oven to 400°F (200°C). Place the diced sweet potatoes on a baking sheet, drizzle with olive oil, and sprinkle with cumin, chili powder, paprika, salt, and pepper. Toss to coat evenly. Roast in the

preheated oven for 20-25 minutes, or until the sweet potatoes are tender and lightly browned.

2. **Prepare Black Beans:** In a small saucepan, heat the black beans over medium heat until warmed through. You can add a pinch of salt and cumin for extra flavor if desired. Once heated, remove from heat and set aside.

3. **Warm Tortillas:** Heat the tortillas in a dry skillet over medium heat for about 30 seconds on each side until warm and pliable. Alternatively, you can warm them in the microwave wrapped in a damp paper towel.

4. **Assemble Tacos:** Spoon a portion of the roasted sweet potatoes and black beans onto each warm tortilla. Add your desired toppings such as diced avocado, salsa, shredded lettuce, and chopped cilantro.

5. **Serve:** Squeeze fresh lime juice over the tacos and serve immediately.

Benefits:

- **Nutrient-Rich:** Sweet potatoes are rich in vitamins A and C, fiber, and various antioxidants, making them a nutritious addition to your diet.

- **Protein and Fiber:** Black beans are an excellent source of plant-based protein and fiber, which can help keep you feeling full and satisfied.

- **Heart-Healthy:** Both sweet potatoes and black beans contain nutrients that support heart health, such as potassium and antioxidants.

- **Vegetarian-Friendly:** This recipe is vegetarian and can easily be made vegan by omitting any dairy-based toppings.

- **Customizable:** Feel free to customize the toppings based on your preferences. You can add ingredients like diced tomatoes, jalapeños, or shredded cheese.

- **Quick and Easy:** This recipe comes together quickly, making it perfect for busy weeknights when you need a nutritious meal on the table fast.

- **Family-Friendly:** These tacos are sure to be a hit with the whole family, providing a tasty way to incorporate more vegetables and plant-based protein into your diet.

Spinach and Feta Stuffed Chicken

Ingredients:

- 4 boneless, skinless chicken breasts
- 2 cups fresh spinach leaves
- 1/2 cup crumbled feta cheese
- 2 cloves garlic, minced
- 1 tablespoon olive oil
- Salt and pepper, to taste
- Toothpicks or kitchen twine, for securing

Preparation:

1. **Prepare Chicken:** Preheat your oven to 375°F (190°C). Place each chicken breast between two sheets of plastic wrap and pound with a meat mallet or rolling pin until flattened to about 1/4-inch thickness.

2. **Sauté Spinach and Garlic:** In a skillet, heat olive oil over medium heat. Add minced garlic and sauté for 1 minute until fragrant. Add fresh spinach leaves and cook until wilted, about 2-3 minutes. Remove from heat and let cool slightly.

3. **Stuff Chicken:** Lay the flattened chicken breasts flat on a clean surface. Divide the sautéed spinach evenly among the chicken breasts, spreading it out in the center. Sprinkle crumbled feta cheese over the spinach.

4. **Roll and Secure:** Starting from one end, roll each chicken breast tightly around the spinach and feta filling. Secure with toothpicks or kitchen twine to hold the rolls together.

5. **Season:** Season the outside of the stuffed chicken breasts with salt and pepper to taste.

6. **Bake:** Place the stuffed chicken breasts in a baking dish or on a baking sheet lined with parchment paper. Bake in the preheated oven for 25-30 minutes, or until the chicken is cooked through and the juices run clear.

7. **Rest and Serve:** Remove the stuffed chicken breasts from the oven and let them rest for a few minutes before serving. Optionally, remove the toothpicks or kitchen twine before serving.

Benefits:

- **High Protein:** Chicken breasts are a lean source of protein, which is essential for muscle repair and growth.

- **Leafy Greens:** Spinach is packed with vitamins, minerals, and antioxidants, promoting overall health and well-being.

- **Calcium and Protein:** Feta cheese provides calcium and additional protein, important for bone health and muscle function.

- **Heart-Healthy Fats:** Olive oil used in cooking offers healthy monounsaturated fats, which can help lower cholesterol levels and reduce the risk of heart disease.

- **Low Carb Option:** This recipe is low in carbohydrates, making it suitable for those following a low-carb or ketogenic diet.

- **Versatile:** You can customize the filling by adding ingredients such as sun-dried tomatoes, artichoke hearts, or roasted red peppers for extra flavor and texture.

- **Impressive Presentation:** Spinach and feta stuffed chicken makes for an elegant and delicious main course that's perfect for entertaining or special occasions.

Cauliflower Rice Stir-Fry

Ingredients:

- 1 medium head of cauliflower

- 2 tablespoons sesame oil

- 2 cloves garlic, minced

- 1 small onion, diced

- 1 cup mixed vegetables (such as bell peppers, carrots, snap peas)

- 2 eggs, beaten

- 3 tablespoons soy sauce

- 1 tablespoon rice vinegar

- Salt and pepper, to taste

- Optional toppings: sliced green onions, sesame seeds, chopped peanuts

Preparation:

1. **Prepare Cauliflower Rice:** Cut the cauliflower into florets and pulse in a food processor until it resembles rice grains. Alternatively, you can use a box grater to grate the cauliflower. Set aside.

2. **Stir-Fry Vegetables:** Heat sesame oil in a large skillet or wok over medium-high

heat. Add minced garlic and diced onion, and sauté until fragrant, about 1-2 minutes.

3. **Add Mixed Vegetables:** Add the mixed vegetables to the skillet and stir-fry until they start to soften, about 3-4 minutes.

4. **Cook Cauliflower Rice:** Push the vegetables to the side of the skillet and add the cauliflower rice. Cook, stirring occasionally, until the cauliflower is tender but still slightly crisp, about 4-5 minutes.

5. **Scramble Eggs:** Push the cauliflower rice and vegetables to the side of the skillet again. Pour the beaten eggs into the empty space and scramble until cooked through.

6. **Combine Ingredients:** Once the eggs are cooked, mix everything together in the skillet. Add soy sauce and rice vinegar, and season with salt and pepper to taste. Stir well to combine all the flavors.

7. **Serve:** Remove the cauliflower rice stir-fry from heat and transfer to serving plates. Garnish with sliced green onions,

sesame seeds, and chopped peanuts if desired. Serve hot.

Benefits:

- **Low in Carbohydrates:** Cauliflower rice is a low-carb alternative to traditional rice, making this stir-fry suitable for low-carb or ketogenic diets.

- **High in Fiber:** Cauliflower is a good source of dietary fiber, which is important for digestive health and promoting feelings of fullness.

- **Rich in Vitamins and Minerals:** Cauliflower is packed with vitamins and minerals, including vitamin C, vitamin K, folate, and potassium.

- **Versatile:** You can customize this stir-fry by adding your favorite vegetables, protein sources (such as tofu or chicken), or additional seasonings to suit your taste preferences.

- **Quick and Easy:** This recipe comes together quickly and is perfect for busy weeknights when you want a healthy meal on the table fast.

- **Light and Healthy:** Cauliflower rice stir-fry is light, healthy, and packed with flavor, making it a great option for those looking to eat lighter or incorporate more vegetables into their diet.

Eggplant and Tomato Bake

Ingredients:

- 2 medium eggplants, sliced into 1/2-inch rounds
- 2 large tomatoes, sliced into 1/4-inch rounds
- 1/2 cup breadcrumbs
- 1/4 cup grated Parmesan cheese
- 2 cloves garlic, minced
- 2 tablespoons fresh basil, chopped
- 2 tablespoons olive oil
- Salt and pepper, to taste

Preparation:

1. **Preheat Oven:** Preheat your oven to 375°F (190°C). Lightly grease a baking dish with olive oil.

2. **Prepare Eggplant:** Place the sliced eggplants in a colander and sprinkle with salt. Let them sit for about 15-20 minutes to release excess moisture. Rinse the eggplant slices and pat them dry with paper towels.

3. **Layer Eggplant and Tomato:** Arrange half of the eggplant slices in the bottom of the prepared baking dish. Top with half of the sliced tomatoes. Repeat the layers with the remaining eggplant and tomato slices.

4. **Prepare Topping:** In a small bowl, combine breadcrumbs, grated Parmesan cheese, minced garlic, chopped basil, olive oil, salt, and pepper. Mix well to combine.

5. **Top with Breadcrumb Mixture:** Sprinkle the breadcrumb mixture evenly over the top of the layered eggplant and tomato slices.

6. **Bake:** Cover the baking dish with aluminum foil and bake in the preheated oven for 25-30 minutes. Then, remove the foil and continue baking for an additional 10-15 minutes, or until the breadcrumbs are golden brown and the vegetables are tender.

7. **Serve:** Remove the eggplant and tomato bake from the oven and let it cool for a few minutes before serving. Garnish with additional fresh basil if desired.

Benefits:

- **Rich in Antioxidants:** Eggplant and tomatoes are both rich in antioxidants, including vitamins C and E, which help protect cells from damage caused by free radicals.

- **Low in Calories:** This dish is low in calories but high in nutrient density, making it a great option for those looking to maintain a healthy weight.

- **High in Fiber:** Eggplant is a good source of dietary fiber, which is important for digestive health and promoting feelings of fullness.

- **Heart-Healthy:** Olive oil used in this recipe provides heart-healthy monounsaturated fats, which can help lower cholesterol levels and reduce the risk of heart disease.

- **Versatile:** This eggplant and tomato bake can be served as a side dish or a main course. It pairs well with grilled chicken, fish, or tofu.

- **Easy to Make:** This recipe is simple and easy to prepare, making it perfect for busy weeknights or as a healthy option for entertaining guests.

- **Vegetarian and Gluten-Free:** This dish is vegetarian and can be made gluten-free by using gluten-free breadcrumbs or omitting the breadcrumbs altogether.

Greek Yogurt Parfait

Ingredients:

- 1 cup Greek yogurt

- 1/2 cup granola

- 1/2 cup mixed berries (such as strawberries, blueberries, raspberries)

- 1 tablespoon honey or maple syrup (optional)

- 1 tablespoon chopped nuts (such as almonds, walnuts) (optional)

Preparation:

1. **Layer Yogurt:** Start by spooning a layer of Greek yogurt into the bottom of a glass or bowl.

2. **Add Granola:** Sprinkle a layer of granola over the yogurt.

3. **Layer Berries:** Add a layer of mixed berries on top of the granola.

4. **Repeat Layers:** Repeat the layers of yogurt, granola, and berries until the glass or bowl is filled or all ingredients are used.

5. **Drizzle with Honey:** Optionally, drizzle honey or maple syrup over the top of the parfait for added sweetness.

6. **Garnish with Nuts:** Optionally, sprinkle chopped nuts over the top of the parfait for added crunch and flavor.

7. **Serve:** Serve the Greek yogurt parfait immediately as a nutritious breakfast, snack, or dessert option.

Benefits:

- **High in Protein:** Greek yogurt is rich in protein, which helps keep you feeling full and satisfied throughout the day.

- **Rich in Probiotics:** Greek yogurt contains probiotics, beneficial bacteria that support digestive health and boost the immune system.

- **Antioxidant-Rich:** Berries are packed with antioxidants, vitamins, and minerals, which help protect cells from damage caused by free radicals.

- **Source of Fiber:** Granola provides dietary fiber, which supports digestive health and promotes feelings of fullness.

- **Customizable:** This recipe is highly customizable. You can use your favorite fruits, nuts, and toppings to create a parfait that suits your taste preferences.

- **Quick and Easy:** Greek yogurt parfait is quick and easy to assemble, making it a perfect option for busy mornings or as a healthy snack on the go.

- **Versatile:** Greek yogurt parfait can be enjoyed as a breakfast option, snack, or even a light dessert. It's a versatile dish that can be enjoyed at any time of day.

- **Nutrient-Dense:** This parfait is packed with essential nutrients, including protein, vitamins, minerals, and antioxidants, making it a nutritious and satisfying option for any meal or snack.

Zucchini Noodles with Pesto

Ingredients:

- 4 medium zucchinis
- 1 cup fresh basil leaves
- 1/4 cup pine nuts
- 2 cloves garlic, minced
- 1/4 cup grated Parmesan cheese
- 1/4 cup extra virgin olive oil
- Salt and pepper, to taste
- Optional toppings: cherry tomatoes, grated Parmesan cheese, chopped basil

Preparation:

1. **Prepare Zucchini Noodles:** Using a spiralizer or vegetable peeler, create zucchini noodles by cutting the zucchinis into thin strips. Set aside.

2. **Make Pesto:** In a food processor, combine fresh basil leaves, pine nuts, minced garlic, grated Parmesan cheese, and a pinch of salt and pepper. Pulse until the ingredients are finely chopped.

3. **Add Olive Oil:** With the food processor running, slowly drizzle in the extra virgin olive oil until the pesto reaches a smooth consistency. Taste and adjust seasoning if necessary.

4. **Cook Zucchini Noodles:** Heat a large skillet over medium heat. Add the zucchini noodles and cook for 2-3 minutes, tossing occasionally, until they are just tender but still slightly crisp.

5. **Combine with Pesto:** Add the prepared pesto to the skillet with the zucchini noodles. Toss gently to coat the noodles evenly with the pesto.

6. **Serve:** Remove the zucchini noodles with pesto from the heat and transfer to serving plates. Garnish with optional toppings such as cherry tomatoes, grated Parmesan cheese, and chopped basil.

7. **Enjoy:** Serve immediately as a light and flavorful meal or side dish.

Benefits:

- **Low in Carbohydrates:** Zucchini noodles are a low-carb alternative to traditional pasta, making this dish suitable for low-carb or ketogenic diets.

- **Rich in Vitamins and Minerals:** Zucchinis are packed with vitamins and minerals, including vitamin C, vitamin A, potassium, and folate, which support overall health and well-being.

- **Healthy Fats:** Pine nuts and extra virgin olive oil provide healthy monounsaturated fats, which are beneficial for heart health and can help reduce inflammation.

- **Antioxidants:** Basil is rich in antioxidants, including flavonoids and polyphenols, which help protect cells from damage caused by free radicals.

- **Quick and Easy:** This recipe comes together quickly and is perfect for busy weeknights when you want a healthy meal on the table fast.

- **Versatile:** You can customize this dish by adding additional ingredients such as cherry tomatoes, grilled chicken, or shrimp for extra protein and flavor.

- **Nutrient-Dense:** Zucchini noodles with pesto is a nutrient-dense dish that provides essential nutrients, including vitamins, minerals, fiber, and healthy fats, making it a nutritious and satisfying option for any meal.

Quinoa Stuffed Bell Peppers

Ingredients:

- 4 large bell peppers (any color)

- 1 cup quinoa, rinsed

- 2 cups vegetable broth or water

- 1 tablespoon olive oil

- 1 small onion, diced

- 2 cloves garlic, minced

- 1 medium carrot, diced

- 1 medium zucchini, diced

- 1 cup canned black beans, drained and rinsed

- 1 cup corn kernels (fresh, frozen, or canned)

- 1 teaspoon ground cumin

- 1 teaspoon paprika

- Salt and pepper, to taste

- 1 cup shredded cheese (cheddar, mozzarella, or your favorite cheese)

- Fresh cilantro or parsley, chopped (optional, for garnish)

Preparation:

1. **Preheat Oven:** Preheat your oven to 375°F (190°C). Grease a baking dish large enough to fit the bell peppers.

2. **Prepare Quinoa:** In a saucepan, combine quinoa and vegetable broth or water. Bring to a boil, then reduce heat to low, cover, and simmer for 15-20 minutes, or until quinoa is cooked and liquid is absorbed. Remove from heat and let It sit covered for 5 minutes. Fluff with a fork and set aside.

3. **Prepare Bell Peppers:** Cut the tops off the bell peppers and remove the seeds and membranes. If needed, trim the bottoms slightly so that they can stand upright in the baking dish. Place the bell peppers in the prepared baking dish.

4. **Sauté Vegetables:** In a large skillet, heat olive oil over medium heat. Add diced onion and minced garlic, and sauté until fragrant, about 2-3 minutes. Add diced carrot and zucchini, and cook for another 5 minutes, or until the vegetables are softened.

5. **Add Quinoa Mixture:** Stir in cooked quinoa, black beans, corn kernels, ground cumin, paprika, salt, and pepper. Cook for an additional 2-3 minutes to allow the flavors to meld together.

6. **Stuff Bell Peppers:** Spoon the quinoa mixture evenly into the hollowed-out bell peppers, pressing down gently to pack the filling.

7. **Bake:** Sprinkle shredded cheese over the stuffed bell peppers. Cover the baking dish with aluminum foil and bake in the preheated oven for 25-30 minutes. Then, remove the foil and bake for an additional 10-15 minutes, or until the bell peppers are tender and the cheese is melted and bubbly.

8. **Serve:** Remove the quinoa stuffed bell peppers from the oven and let them cool for a few minutes before serving. Garnish with chopped fresh cilantro or parsley if desired.

Benefits:

- **High in Protein:** Quinoa is a complete protein, providing all nine essential amino acids, making this dish suitable for vegetarians and vegans.

- **Rich in Fiber:** Bell peppers, quinoa, black beans, and vegetables are all high in fiber, which supports digestive health and helps keep you feeling full and satisfied.

- **Packed with Vitamins and Minerals:** Bell peppers are rich in vitamins A and C, while quinoa provides iron, magnesium, and manganese, contributing to overall health and well-being.

- **Low in Calories:** This dish is relatively low in calories but high in nutrient density, making it a nutritious and satisfying option for any meal.

- **Versatile:** You can customize this recipe by using your favorite vegetables, beans, or grains, and adjust the seasonings according to your taste preferences.

- **Make-Ahead Option:** Quinoa stuffed bell peppers can be assembled ahead of time and stored in the refrigerator until ready to bake, making them perfect for meal prep or entertaining guests.

- **Gluten-Free:** This dish is naturally gluten-free, making it suitable for those with gluten sensitivities or celiac disease.

Vegetable Stir-Fry with Tofu

Ingredients:

- 14 oz (400g) firm tofu, pressed and cubed
- 2 tablespoons soy sauce
- 1 tablespoon sesame oil
- 1 tablespoon cornstarch
- 2 tablespoons vegetable oil
- 2 cloves garlic, minced
- 1 tablespoon grated ginger
- 1 bell pepper, thinly sliced
- 1 cup (150g) snap peas, trimmed
- 1 carrot, julienned
- 1 cup (120g) broccoli florets
- 1 cup (100g) sliced mushrooms
- 2 green onions, sliced
- Cooked rice or noodles, for serving
- Sesame seeds (optional, for garnish)

Preparation:

1. **Marinate Tofu:** In a bowl, combine cubed tofu with soy sauce, sesame oil, and

cornstarch. Toss gently to coat the tofu evenly. Let it marinate for 15-30 minutes.

2. **Prepare Aromatics:** In a large skillet or wok, heat vegetable oil over medium-high heat. Add minced garlic and grated ginger. Sauté for about 1 minute until fragrant.

3. **Cook Tofu:** Add the marinated tofu to the skillet. Cook until the tofu is golden brown on all sides, about 5-7 minutes. Remove tofu from the skillet and set aside.

4. **Stir-Fry Vegetables:** In the same skillet, add sliced bell pepper, snap peas, julienned carrot, broccoli florets, and sliced mushrooms. Stir-fry for 4-5 minutes until the vegetables are tender-crisp.

5. **Combine Ingredients:** Return the cooked tofu to the skillet with the vegetables. Add sliced green onions. Stir everything together until heated through.

6. **Season:** Drizzle a little extra soy sauce or sesame oil over the stir-fry if desired. Taste and adjust seasoning as needed.

7. **Serve:** Serve the vegetable stir-fry with tofu hot over cooked rice or noodles. Garnish with sesame seeds if desired.

Benefits:

- **Protein Source:** Tofu provides a plant-based source of protein, making this stir-fry suitable for vegetarians and vegans.

- **Healthy Fats:** Sesame oil offers healthy fats and adds a nutty flavor to the stir-fry.

- **Fiber and Nutrients:** The variety of vegetables in this stir-fry, including bell pepper, snap peas, carrot, broccoli, and mushrooms, provide fiber, vitamins, and minerals essential for overall health.

- **Low in Calories:** This dish is low in calories but high in nutrient density, making it suitable for weight management and promoting satiety.

- **Quick and Easy:** Stir-fries come together quickly and are perfect for busy weeknights when you want a healthy meal on the table fast.

- **Customizable:** You can easily customize this stir-fry by adding your favorite vegetables or adjusting the seasonings to suit your taste preferences.

- **Versatile:** Serve this vegetable stir-fry with tofu over rice, noodles, or quinoa for a complete meal. Leftovers can be enjoyed for lunch the next day or repurposed into wraps, salads, or grain bowls.

Mediterranean Chickpea Salad

Ingredients:

- 2 cans (15 oz each) chickpeas (garbanzo beans), drained and rinsed

- 1 English cucumber, diced

- 1 pint cherry tomatoes, halved

- 1/2 red onion, thinly sliced

- 1/2 cup Kalamata olives, pitted and halved

- 1/2 cup crumbled feta cheese

- 1/4 cup chopped fresh parsley

- 1/4 cup extra virgin olive oil

- 2 tablespoons lemon juice

- 1 teaspoon dried oregano

- Salt and pepper, to taste

Preparation:

1. **Prepare Chickpeas:** In a large mixing bowl, combine the drained and rinsed chickpeas.

2. **Add Vegetables:** Add diced cucumber, halved cherry tomatoes, thinly sliced red

onion, halved Kalamata olives, and chopped fresh parsley to the bowl with the chickpeas.

3. **Make Dressing:** In a small bowl, whisk together extra virgin olive oil, lemon juice, dried oregano, salt, and pepper to make the dressing.

4. **Combine Ingredients:** Pour the dressing over the chickpea and vegetable mixture in the large mixing bowl. Toss gently to coat all ingredients evenly with the dressing.

5. **Add Feta:** Sprinkle crumbled feta cheese over the salad and toss again gently to combine.

6. **Chill:** Cover the bowl with plastic wrap or transfer the salad to an airtight container. Refrigerate for at least 30 minutes to allow the flavors to meld together.

7. **Serve:** Serve the Mediterranean chickpea salad chilled as a refreshing and nutritious side dish or as a light vegetarian main course.

Benefits:

- **High in Protein:** Chickpeas are a good source of plant-based protein, which is essential for muscle repair and growth.

- **Rich in Fiber:** Chickpeas are also rich in fiber, which supports digestive health and helps keep you feeling full and satisfied.

- **Antioxidant-Rich:** This salad is packed with antioxidant-rich vegetables, including tomatoes, cucumbers, onions, and olives, which help protect cells from damage caused by free radicals.

- **Healthy Fats:** Extra virgin olive oil used in the dressing provides heart-healthy monounsaturated fats, which can help lower cholesterol levels and reduce the risk of heart disease.

- **Calcium Source:** Feta cheese adds calcium to the salad, which is important for bone health.

- **Quick and Easy:** This recipe comes together quickly and is perfect for meal prep or as a last-minute side dish for gatherings or weeknight dinners.

- **Customizable:** You can customize this salad by adding additional ingredients such as bell peppers, artichoke hearts, or fresh herbs according to your taste preferences.

Salmon Avocado Salad

Ingredients:

- 2 salmon fillets (6-8 oz each), skin-on
- 4 cups mixed salad greens (such as spinach, arugula, or lettuce)
- 1 ripe avocado, sliced
- 1 cup cherry tomatoes, halved
- 1/4 red onion, thinly sliced
- 1/4 cup sliced almonds
- 2 tablespoons chopped fresh dill (optional, for garnish)
- 2 tablespoons extra virgin olive oil
- 1 tablespoon lemon juice
- Salt and pepper, to taste

Preparation:

1. **Cook Salmon:** Preheat your oven to 400°F (200°C). Place the salmon fillets on a baking sheet lined with parchment paper, skin-side down. Drizzle with olive oil and season with salt and pepper. Bake for 12-15 minutes, or until the salmon is cooked through and flakes easily with a

fork. Remove from the oven and let it cool slightly.

2. **Prepare Salad Greens:** In a large salad bowl, add the mixed greens.

3. **Assemble Salad:** Top the mixed greens with sliced avocado, halved cherry tomatoes, thinly sliced red onion, and sliced almonds.

4. **Flake Salmon:** Once the salmon has cooled slightly, use a fork to flake the salmon into bite-sized pieces. Add the flaked salmon to the salad bowl.

5. **Make Dressing:** In a small bowl, whisk together extra virgin olive oil, lemon juice, salt, and pepper to make the dressing.

6. **Dress Salad:** Drizzle the dressing over the salad ingredients in the bowl.

7. **Toss and Serve:** Gently toss all the ingredients together until evenly coated with the dressing.

8. **Garnish:** Optionally, garnish the salad with chopped fresh dill for added flavor and freshness.

9. **Serve:** Serve the salmon avocado salad immediately as a nutritious and satisfying main course.

Benefits:

- **Rich in Omega-3 Fatty Acids:** Salmon is a rich source of omega-3 fatty acids, which are beneficial for heart health and brain function.

- **High in Protein:** Salmon is also high in protein, which is essential for muscle repair and growth.

- **Healthy Fats:** Avocado provides healthy monounsaturated fats, which can help lower cholesterol levels and reduce the risk of heart disease.

- **Fiber and Nutrients:** The mixed greens, cherry tomatoes, red onion, and almonds in this salad provide fiber, vitamins, and minerals essential for overall health and well-being.

- **Low in Carbohydrates:** This salad is low in carbohydrates, making it suitable for low-carb or ketogenic diets.

- **Quick and Easy:** This recipe comes together quickly and is perfect for a healthy lunch or dinner option on busy weeknights.

- **Customizable:** You can customize this salad by adding additional ingredients such as cucumbers, bell peppers, or crumbled feta cheese according to your taste preferences.

- **Nutrient-Dense:** This salad is packed with essential nutrients, including protein, healthy fats, vitamins, and minerals, making it a nutritious and satisfying option for any meal.

Turmeric Ginger Lentil Soup

Ingredients:

- 1 cup dried red lentils, rinsed
- 1 onion, diced
- 2 carrots, diced
- 2 celery stalks, diced
- 3 cloves garlic, minced
- 1 tablespoon fresh ginger, grated
- 1 tablespoon ground turmeric
- 6 cups vegetable broth
- 1 can (14 oz) diced tomatoes
- 1 teaspoon ground cumin
- 1 teaspoon ground coriander
- Salt and pepper, to taste
- 2 tablespoons olive oil
- Fresh cilantro or parsley, chopped (for garnish)
- Lemon wedges (for serving)

Preparation:

1. **Sauté Aromatics:** Heat olive oil in a large pot over medium heat. Add diced onion, carrots, and celery. Sauté for 5-7 minutes, or until vegetables are softened.

2. **Add Spices:** Add minced garlic, grated ginger, ground turmeric, ground cumin, and ground coriander to the pot. Cook for another 1-2 minutes until fragrant.

3. **Cook Lentils:** Add rinsed red lentils, vegetable broth, and diced tomatoes to the pot. Stir to combine. Bring the mixture to a boil, then reduce the heat to low and let it simmer for about 20-25 minutes, or until lentils are tender and soup has thickened.

4. **Season:** Season the soup with salt and pepper to taste. Adjust seasoning if necessary.

5. **Blend (Optional):** For a smoother consistency, use an immersion blender to partially blend the soup, leaving some lentils and vegetables whole for texture. Alternatively, transfer a portion of the soup to a blender and blend until smooth, then return it to the pot.

6. **Serve:** Ladle the turmeric ginger lentil soup into bowls. Garnish with fresh chopped cilantro or parsley. Serve with lemon wedges on the side for squeezing over the soup before eating.

Benefits:

- **High in Protein and Fiber:** Lentils are a great source of plant-based protein and fiber, making this soup filling and satisfying.

- **Anti-Inflammatory:** Turmeric and ginger are known for their anti-inflammatory properties, which may help reduce inflammation and promote overall health.

- **Rich in Antioxidants:** Turmeric and tomatoes are both rich in antioxidants, which help protect cells from damage caused by free radicals.

- **Immune-Boosting:** Garlic and ginger have immune-boosting properties, which may help support the immune system and ward off illness.

- **Heart-Healthy:** This soup is low in saturated fat and cholesterol, making it heart-healthy and suitable for those watching their cardiovascular health.

- **Nutrient-Dense:** Packed with vegetables, lentils, and spices, this soup is nutrient-dense and provides a variety of vitamins, minerals, and phytonutrients essential for overall health and well-being.

- **Comforting and Warming:** Perfect for colder days, this turmeric ginger lentil soup is comforting, warming, and nourishing for both the body and soul.

Grilled Lemon Herb Chicken

Ingredients:

- 4 boneless, skinless chicken breasts

- 2 lemons, juiced and zested

- 3 cloves garlic, minced

- 2 tablespoons fresh herbs (such as thyme, rosemary, and oregano), chopped

- 2 tablespoons olive oil

- Salt and pepper, to taste

Preparation:

1. **Marinate Chicken:** In a bowl, combine lemon juice, lemon zest, minced garlic, chopped fresh herbs, olive oil, salt, and pepper. Mix well to create the marinade.

2. **Tenderize Chicken:** Place the chicken breasts between two sheets of plastic wrap and gently pound them with a meat mallet or rolling pin to an even thickness of about 1/2 inch. This helps tenderize the chicken and ensures even cooking.

3. **Marinate Chicken:** Place the chicken breasts in a shallow dish or resealable plastic bag. Pour the marinade over the

chicken, making sure each piece is well coated. Cover or seal the dish/bag and refrigerate for at least 30 minutes, or up to 4 hours, to allow the flavors to infuse.

4. **Preheat Grill:** Preheat your grill to medium-high heat (about 375-400°F or 190-200°C).

5. **Grill Chicken:** Remove the chicken breasts from the marinade and discard any excess marinade. Place the chicken on the preheated grill and cook for 6-8 minutes per side, or until the internal temperature reaches 165°F (75°C) and the chicken is cooked through. Cooking times may vary depending on the thickness of the chicken breasts.

6. **Rest and Serve:** Once cooked, transfer the grilled lemon herb chicken to a plate and let it rest for a few minutes before serving. This allows the juices to redistribute and ensures the chicken remains tender and juicy.

7. **Serve:** Serve the grilled lemon herb chicken hot, garnished with additional fresh herbs and lemon slices if desired.

Benefits:

- **High in Protein:** Chicken breasts are a lean source of protein, essential for muscle repair and growth.

- **Rich in Vitamin C:** Lemons are a rich source of vitamin C, which supports immune function and promotes overall health.

- **Antioxidant-Rich Herbs:** Fresh herbs such as thyme, rosemary, and oregano are rich in antioxidants, which help protect cells from damage caused by free radicals.

- **Heart-Healthy Fats:** Olive oil used in the marinade provides heart-healthy monounsaturated fats, which can help lower cholesterol levels and reduce the risk of heart disease.

- **Low in Carbohydrates:** This grilled chicken recipe is low in carbohydrates, making it suitable for low-carb or ketogenic diets.

- **Quick and Easy:** This recipe comes together quickly and is perfect for a weeknight dinner or weekend barbecue.

- **Versatile:** Grilled lemon herb chicken can be served with a variety of side dishes, such as roasted vegetables, salad, rice, or potatoes, making it a versatile and delicious meal option.

- **Flavorful and Juicy:** Marinating the chicken in a mixture of lemon juice, garlic, and fresh herbs infuses it with flavor and helps keep it tender and juicy during grilling.

CONCLUSION

Congratulations on completing "Fast Feast Protocol Recipes: 28-Day Meal Plans for Effortless Immune Support and Weight Loss Nutrition for Beginners."

Over the past 28 days, you've embarked on a journey to better health and vitality, embracing the power of the Fast Feast Protocol to support your immune system, optimize your nutrition, and achieve your weight loss goals.

As you reflect on your journey, take pride in the progress you've made and the positive changes you've experienced. From increased energy and improved digestion to enhanced mental clarity and a leaner, stronger body, each day has brought you closer to becoming the healthiest version of yourself.

But remember, your journey doesn't end here. The Fast Feast Protocol is not just a 28-day meal plan—it's a sustainable lifestyle approach that you can continue to incorporate into your daily routine for long-term health and wellness.

As you move forward, keep experimenting with new recipes, exploring different fasting protocols, and listening to your body's cues. Remember to practice self-care, prioritize sleep, stay hydrated, and nourish yourself with wholesome, nutrient-rich foods.

And most importantly, be kind to yourself. Remember that progress is not always linear, and setbacks are a natural part of the journey. Celebrate your successes, learn from your challenges, and always keep moving forward with determination and resilience.

Thank you for choosing "Fast Feast Protocol Recipes" as your guide on this transformative journey. May your newfound knowledge and commitment to health continue to serve you well as you embark on the next chapter of your wellness journey.

Here's to a lifetime of vibrant health, happiness, and vitality!

www.ingramcontent.com/pod-product-compliance
Lightning Source LLC
Chambersburg PA
CBHW071149280726
48660CB00020B/652